This Book Belongs To:

_____

Color Test Page

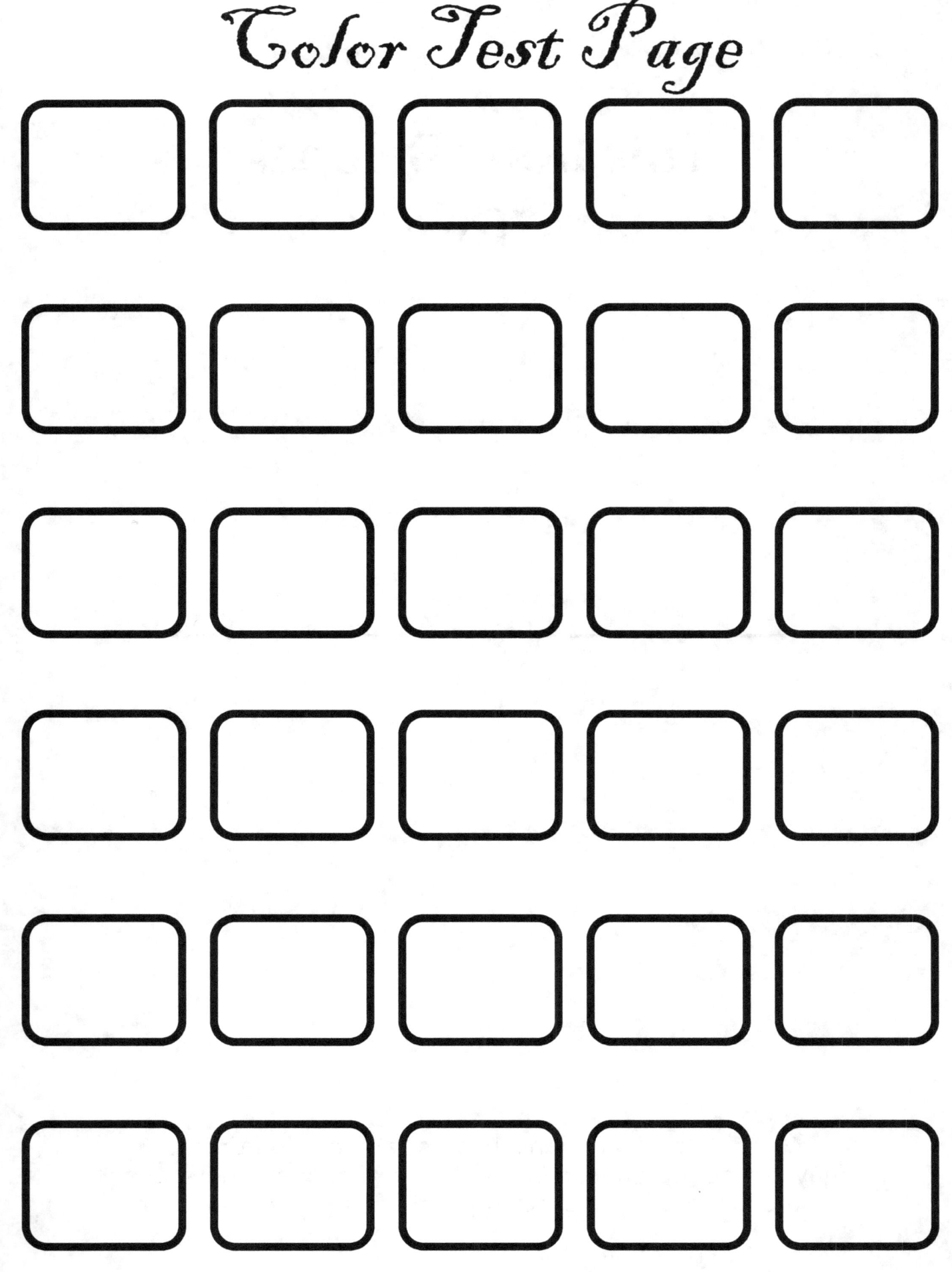

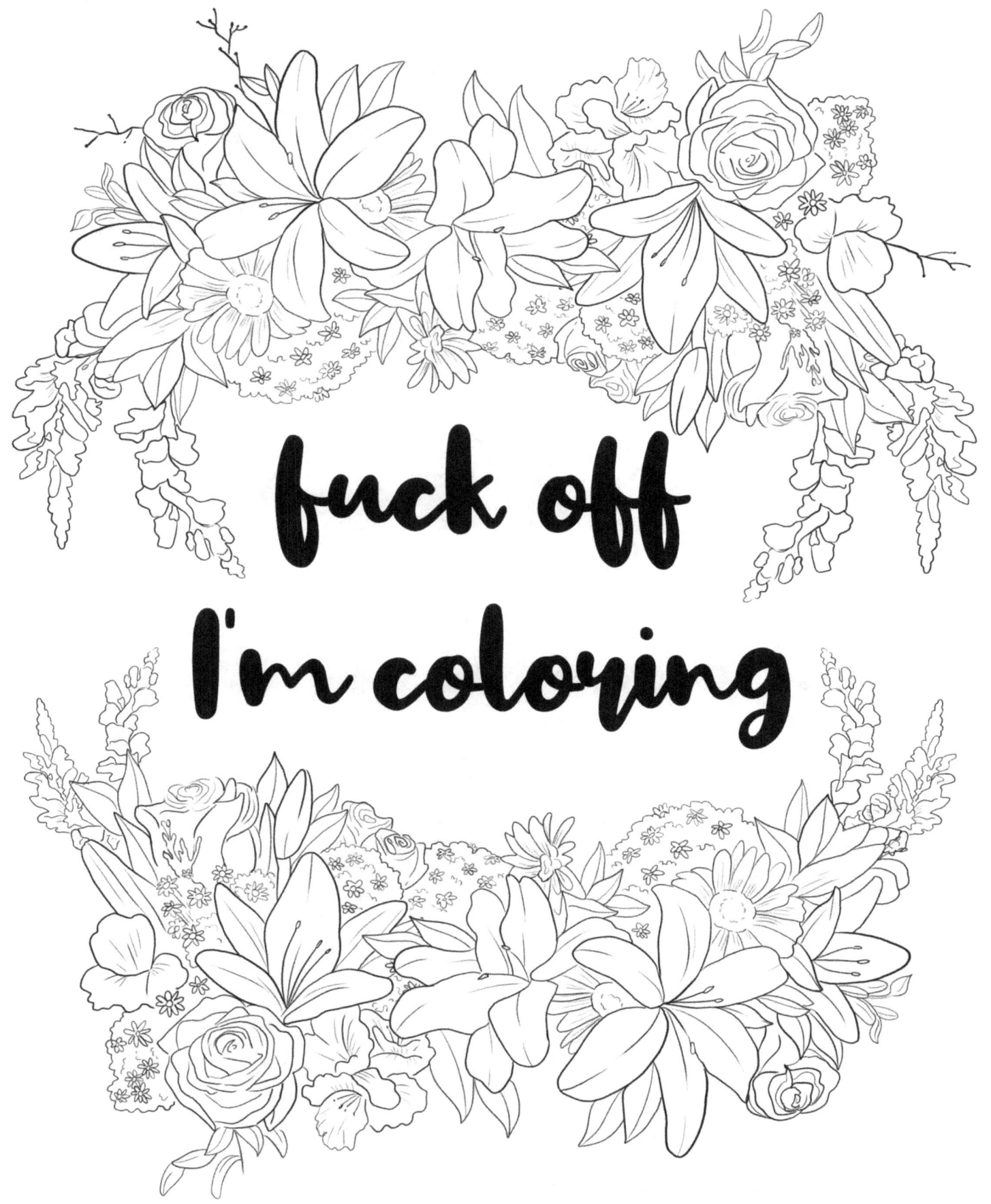

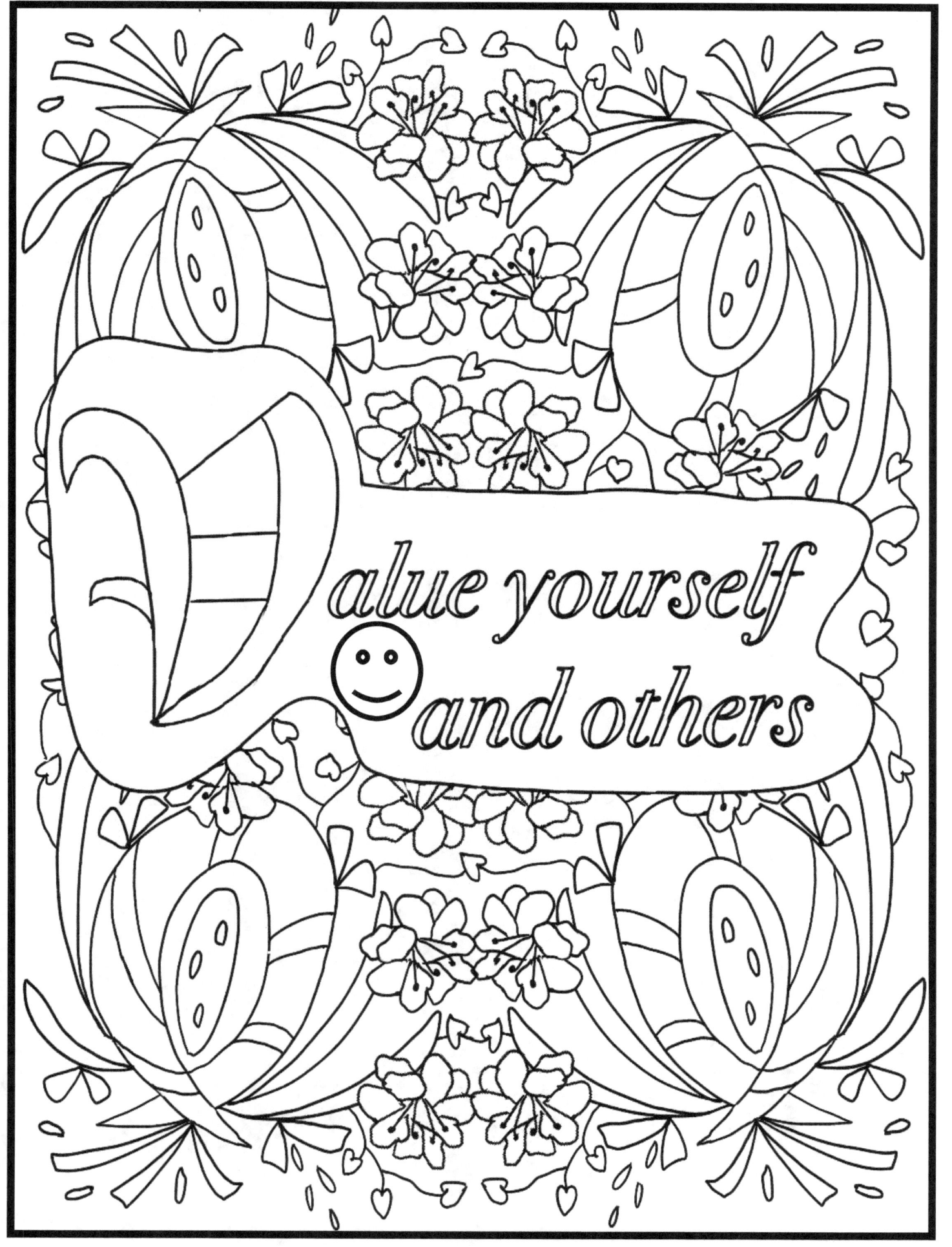

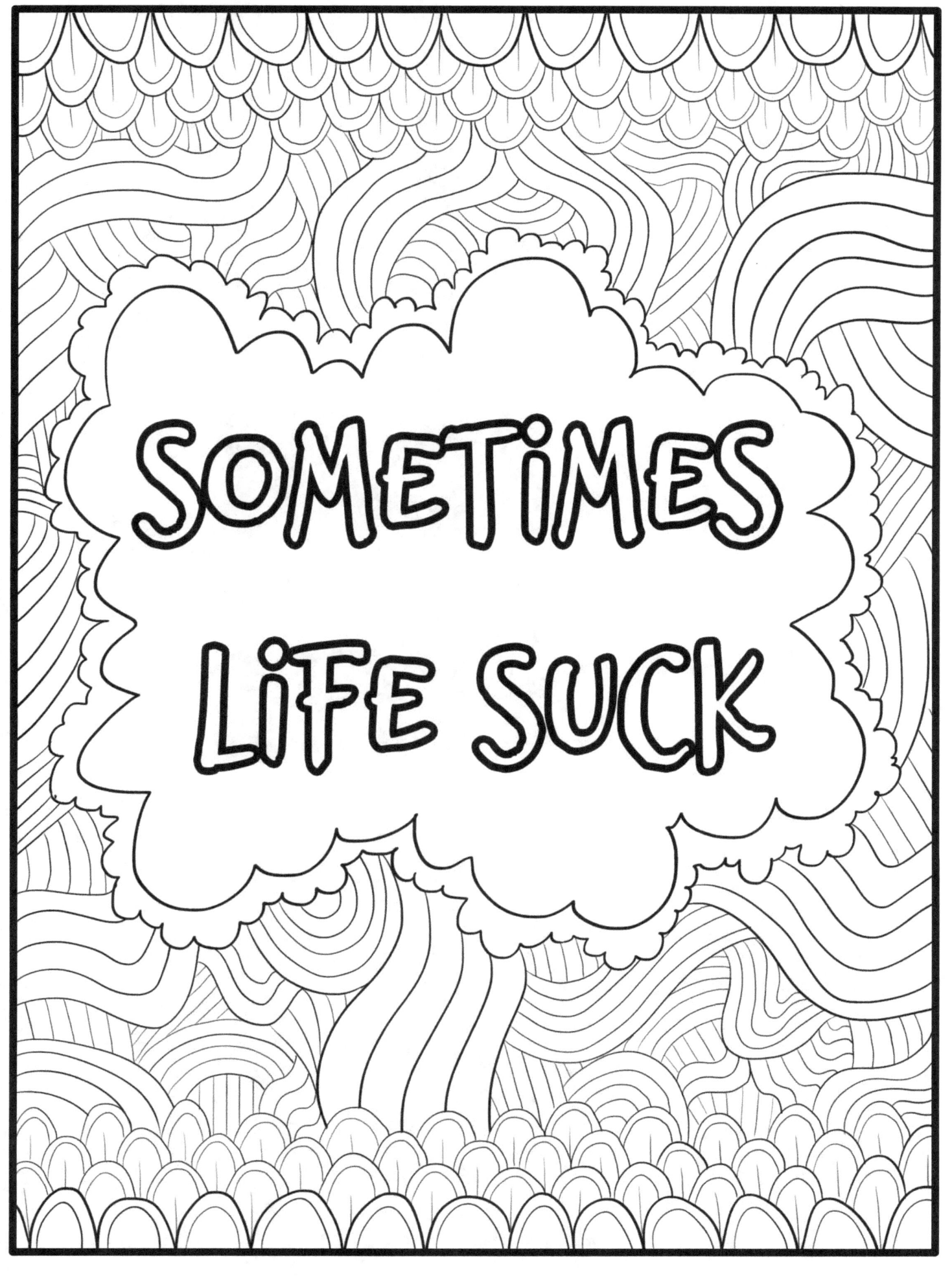

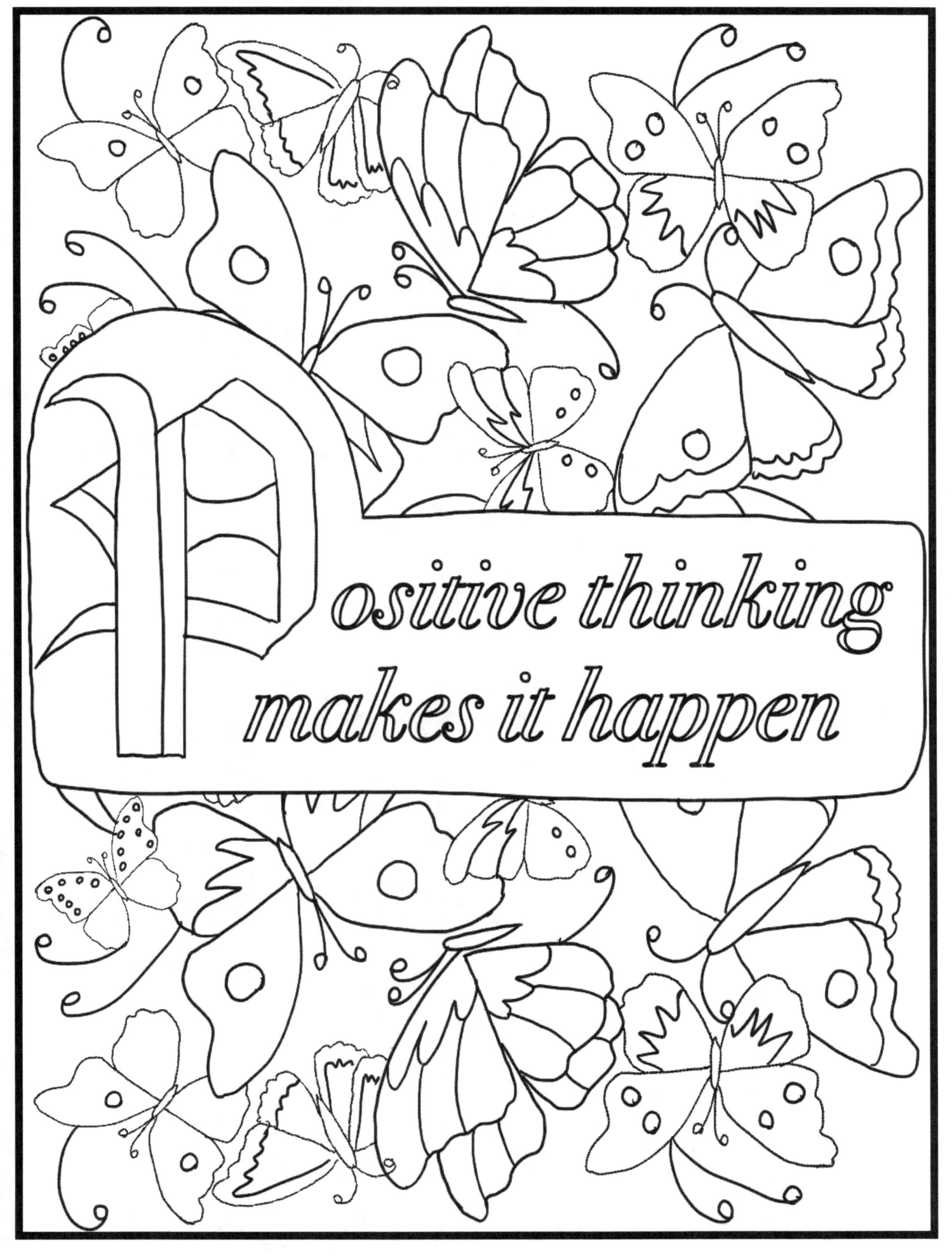

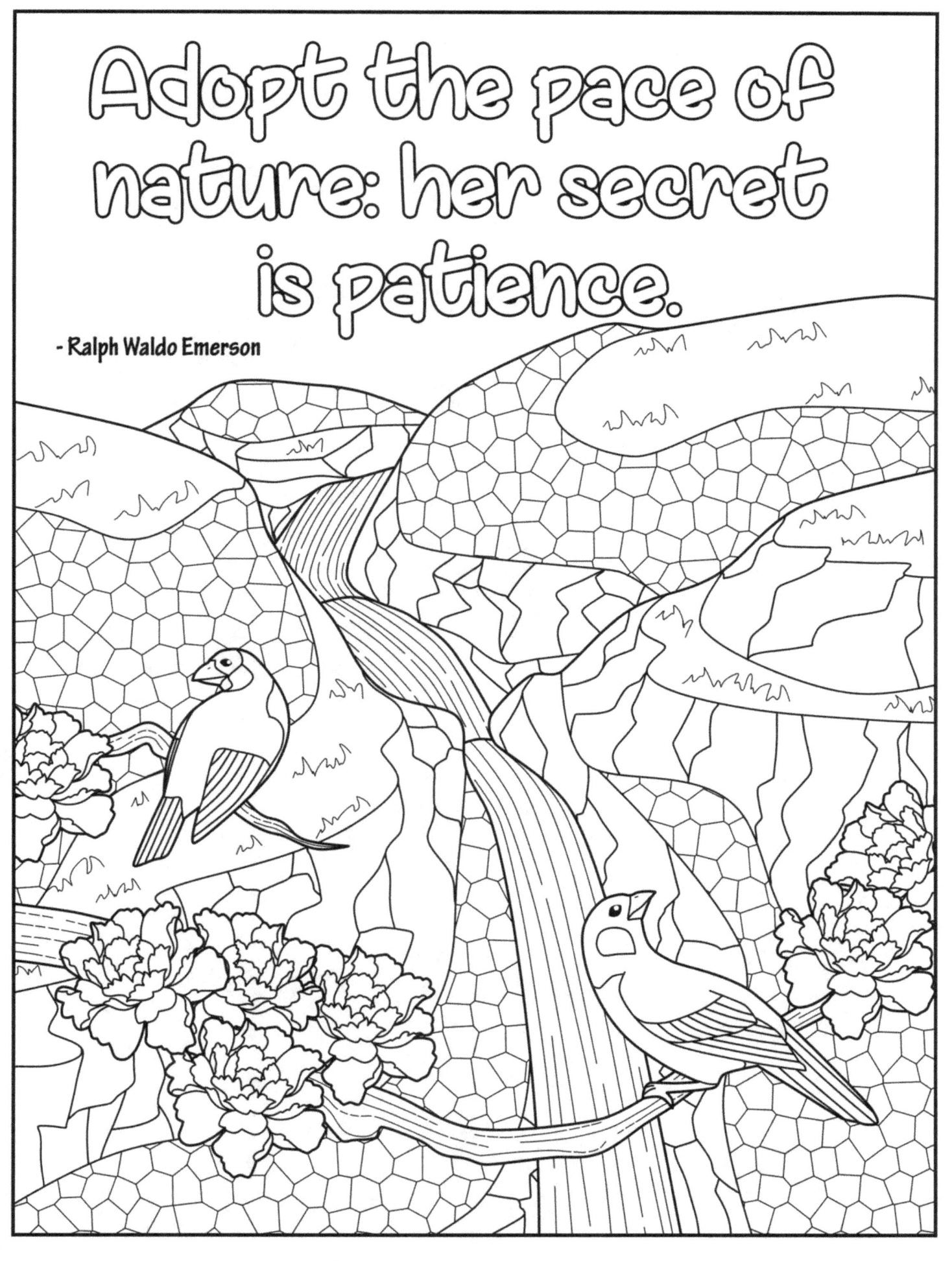

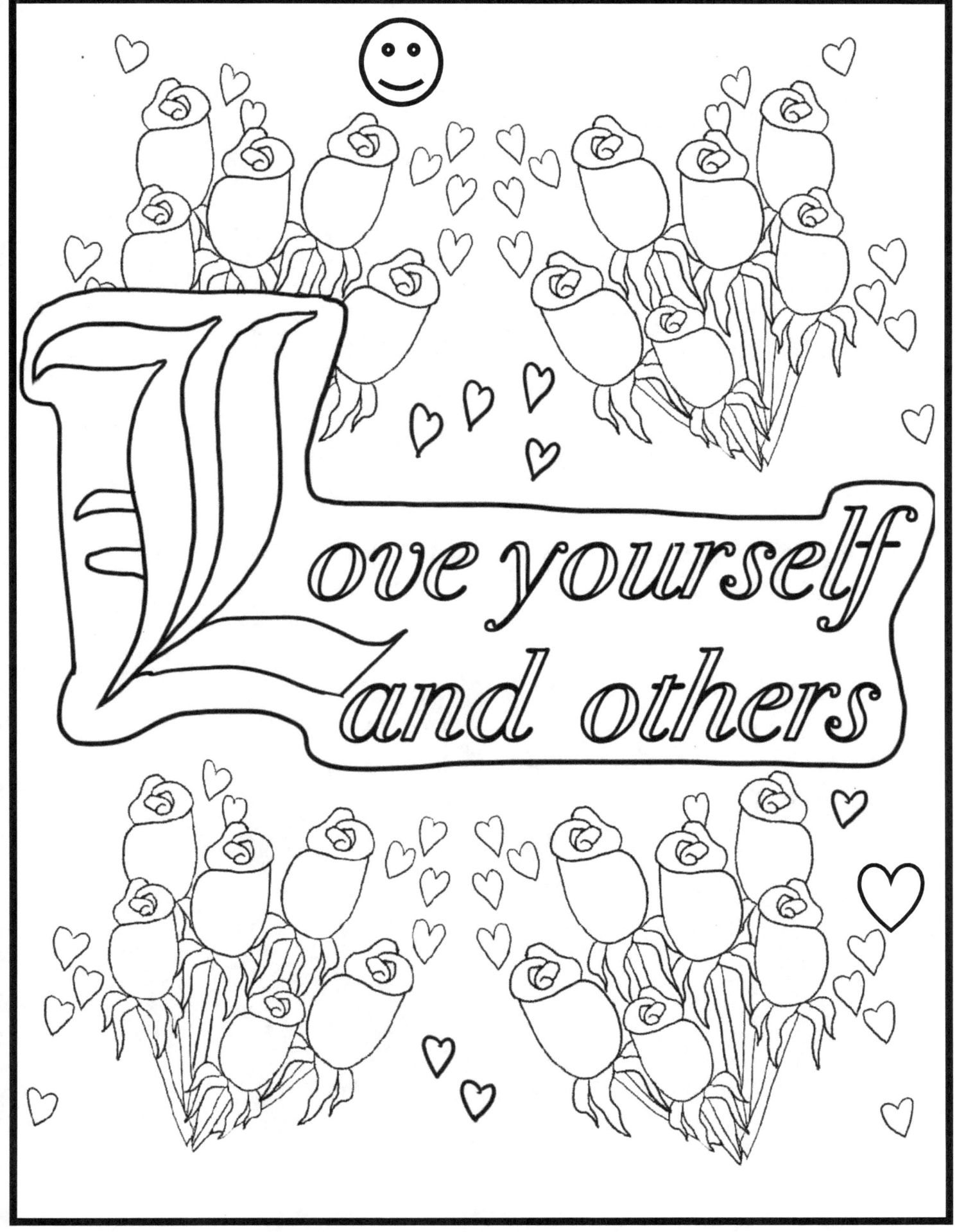

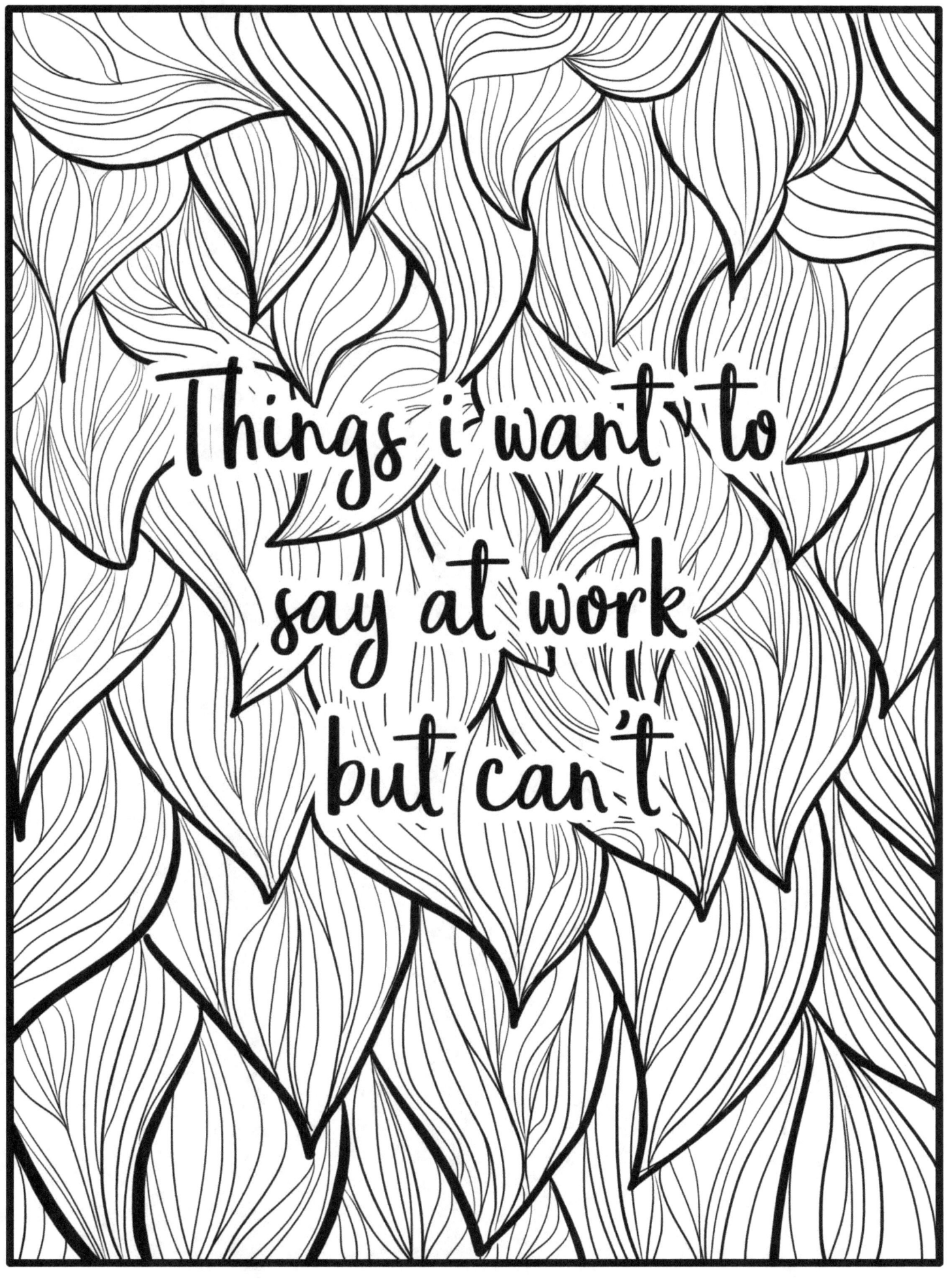

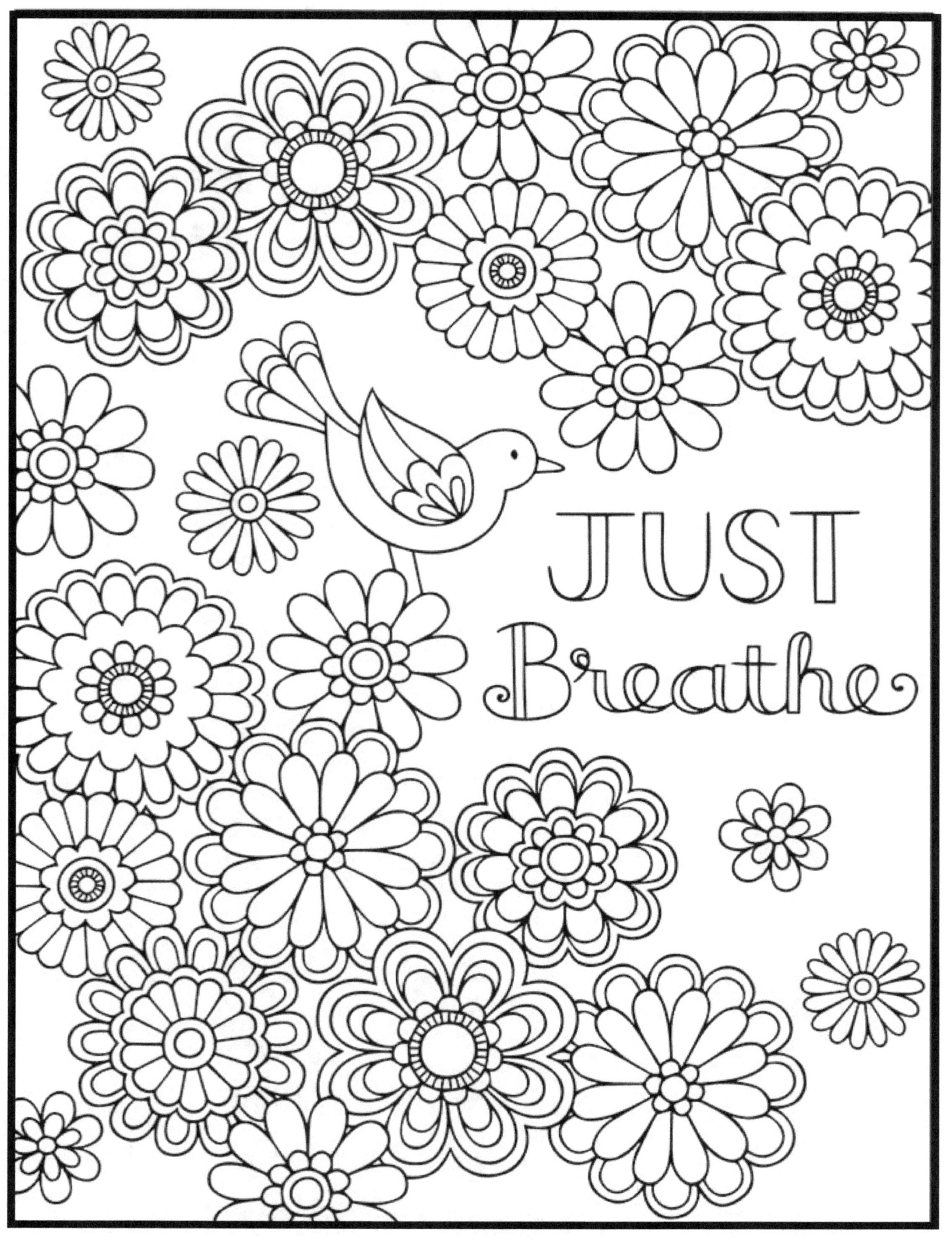

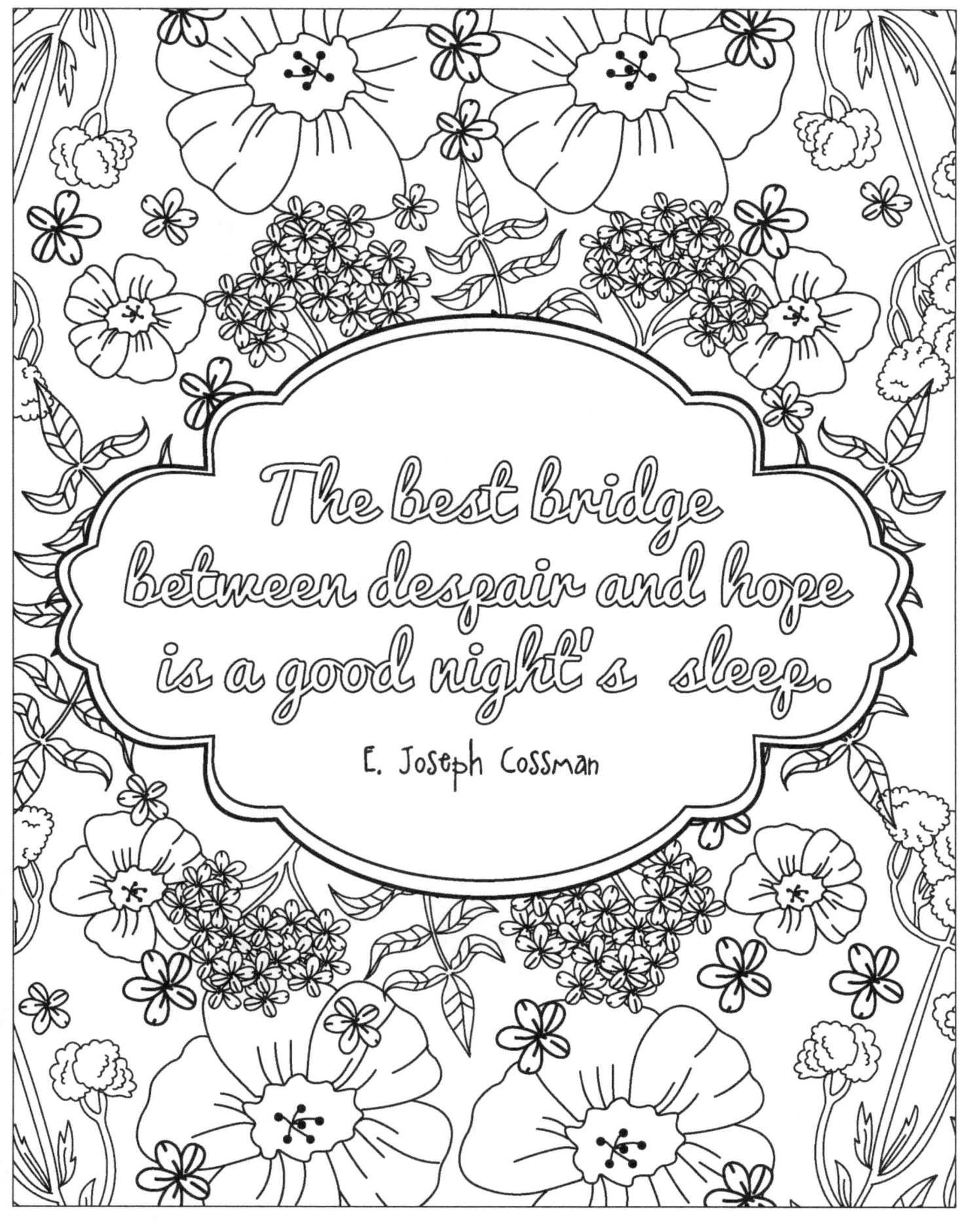

The best bridge between despair and hope is a good night's sleep.

E. Joseph Cossman

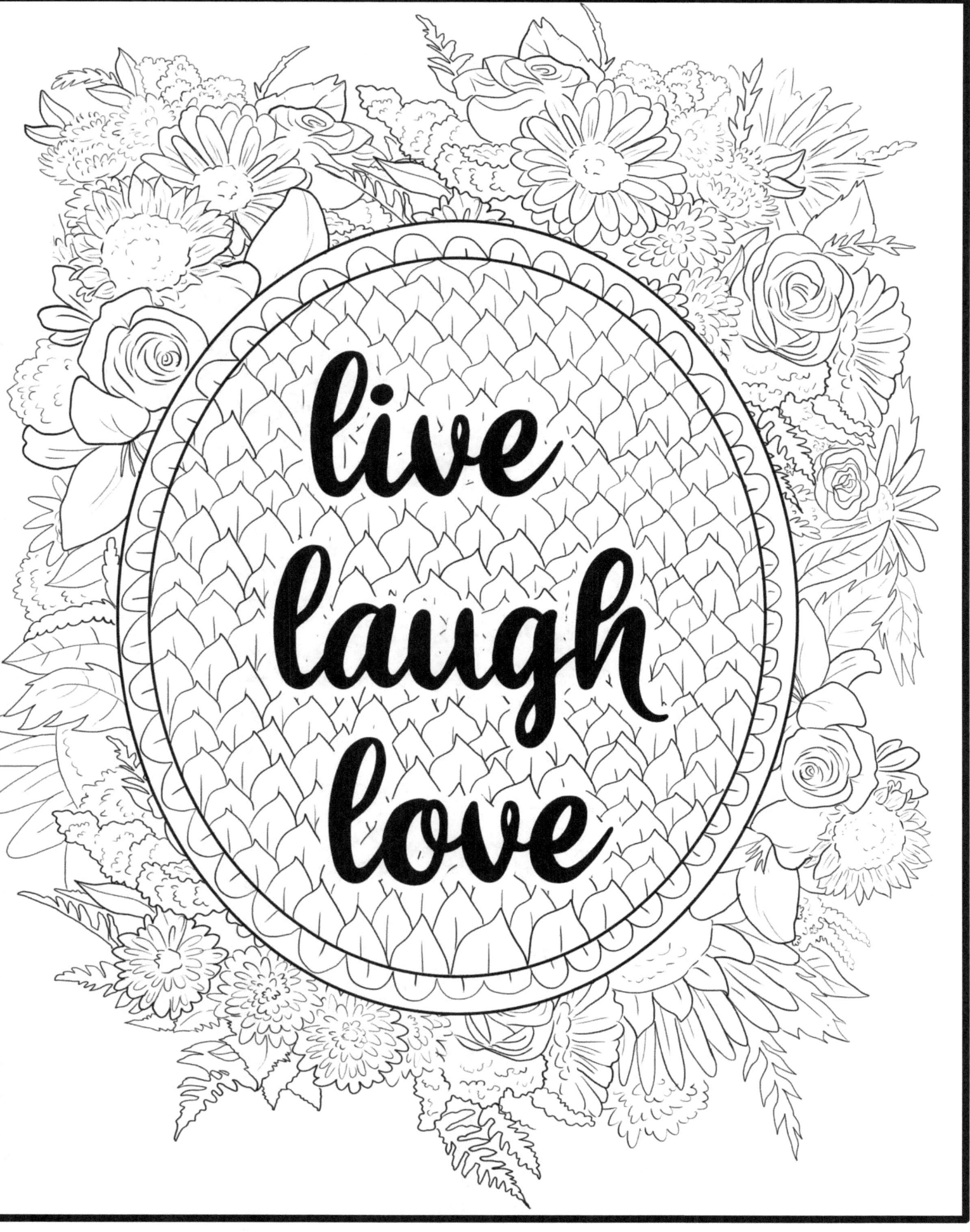

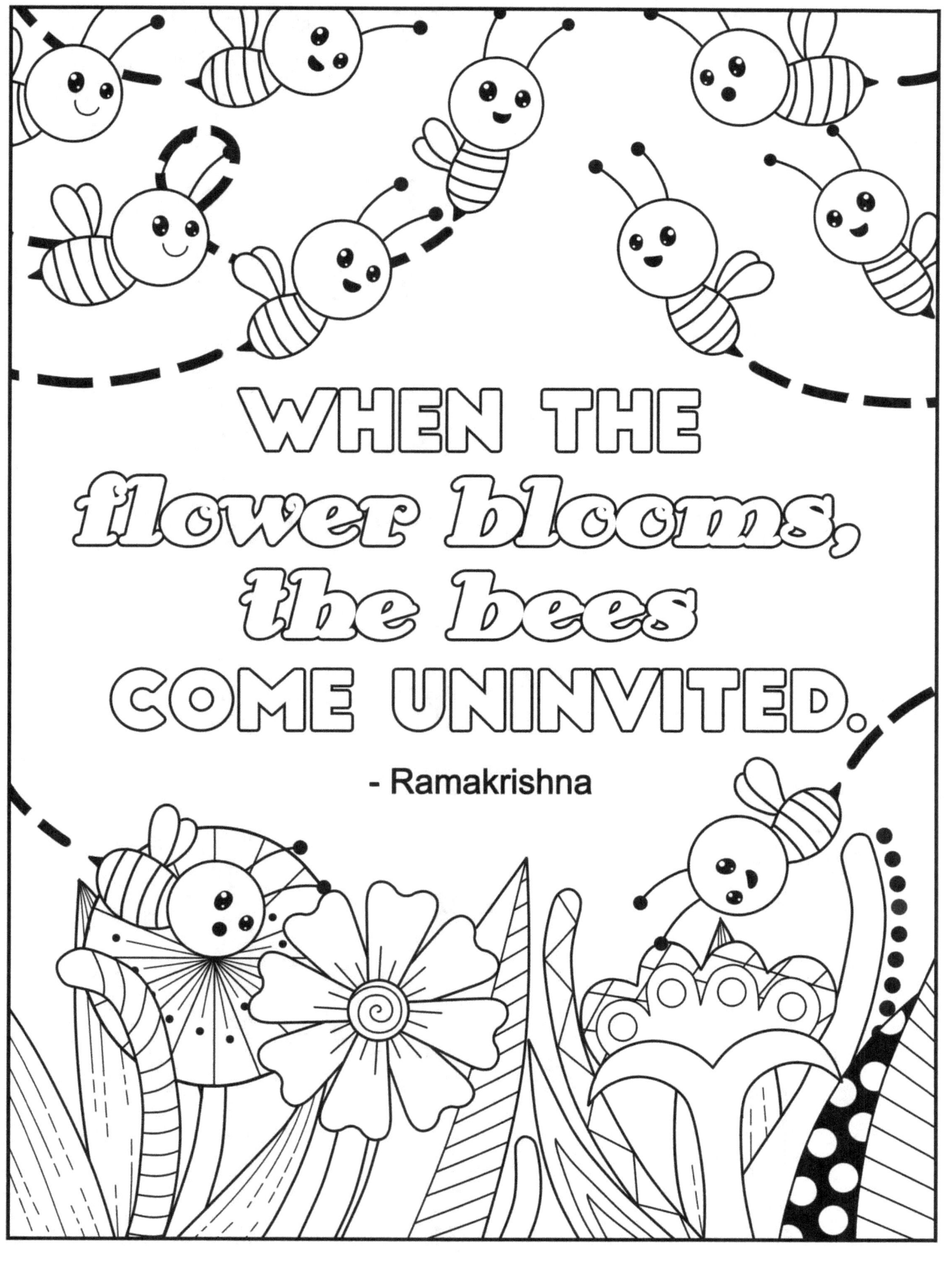

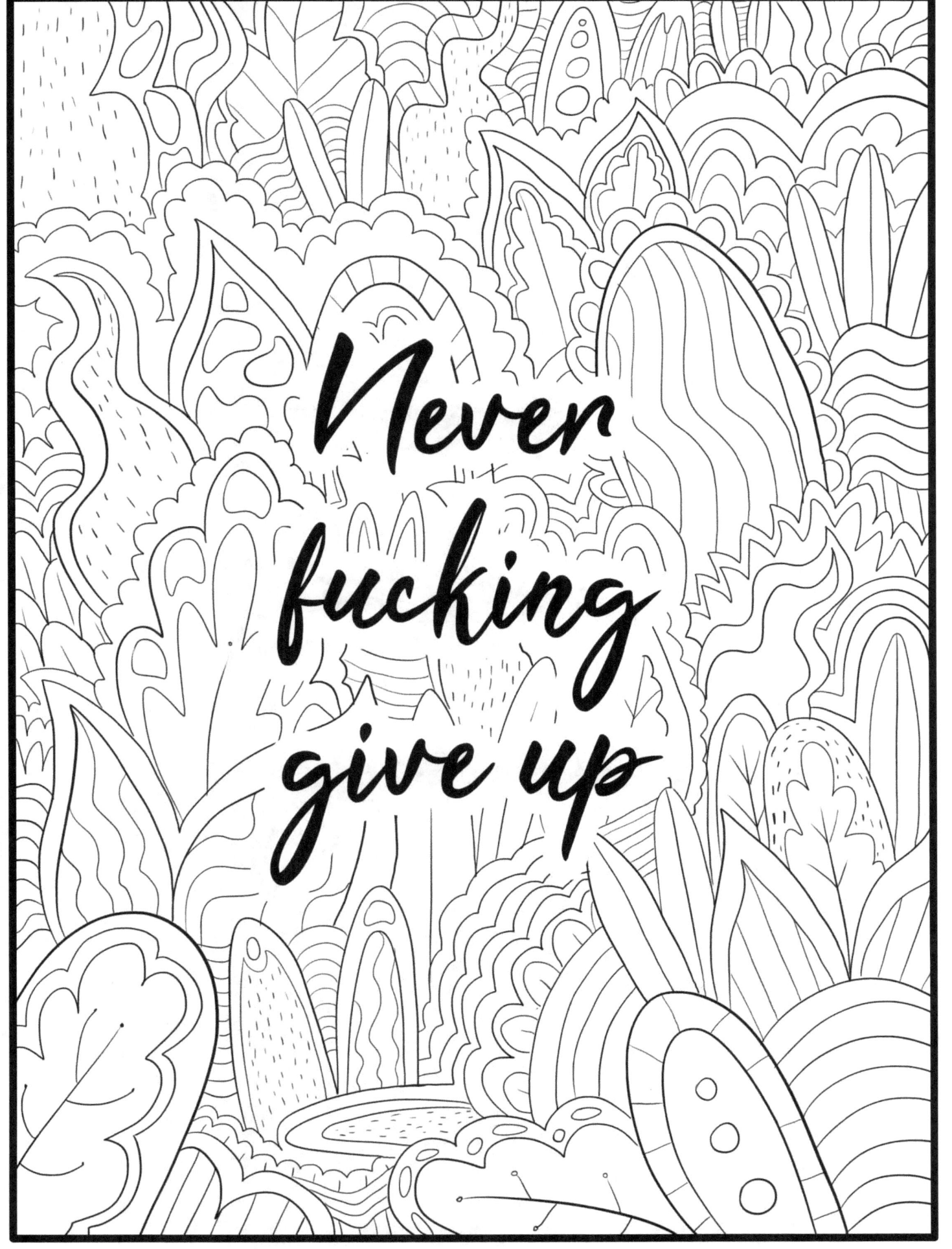

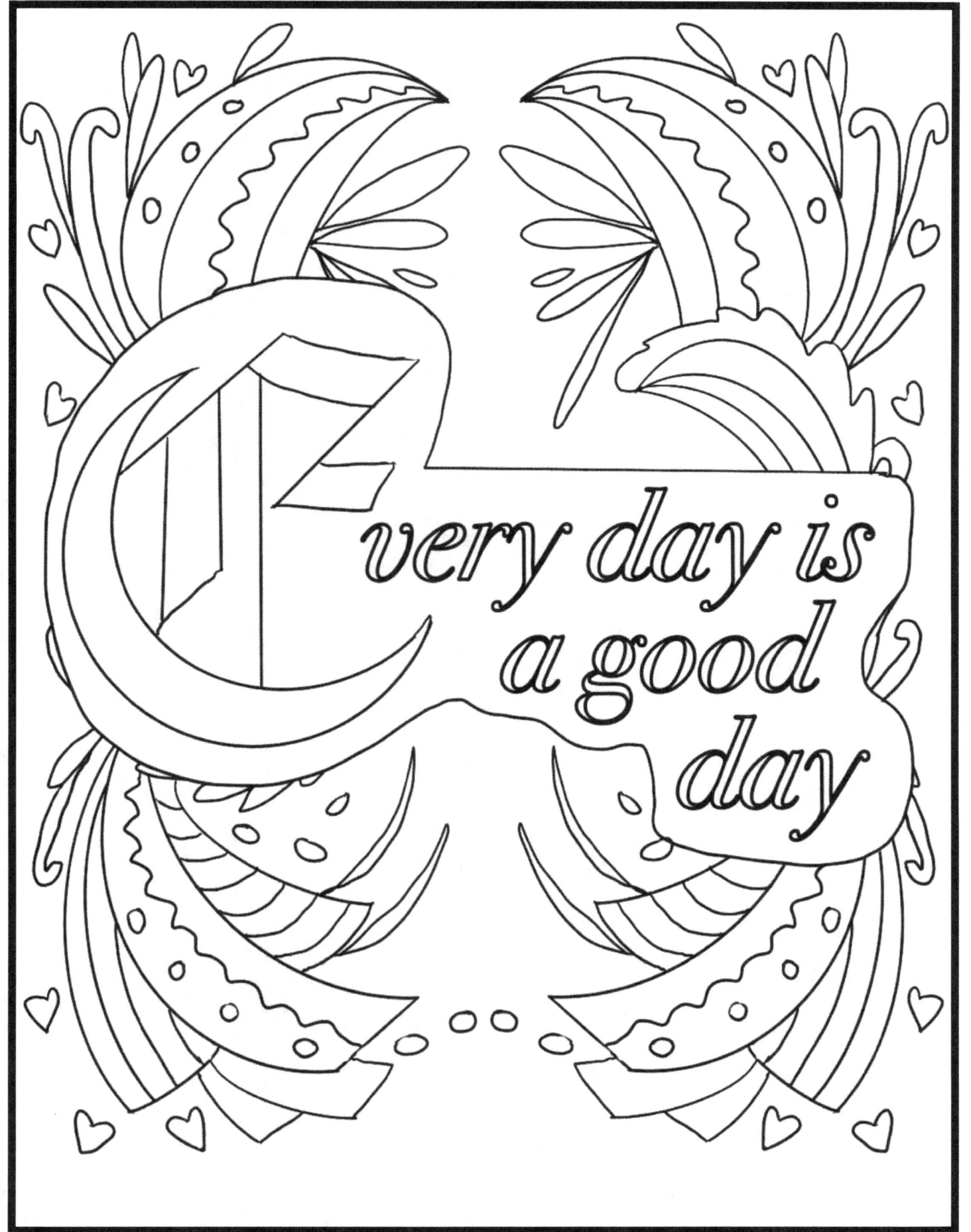

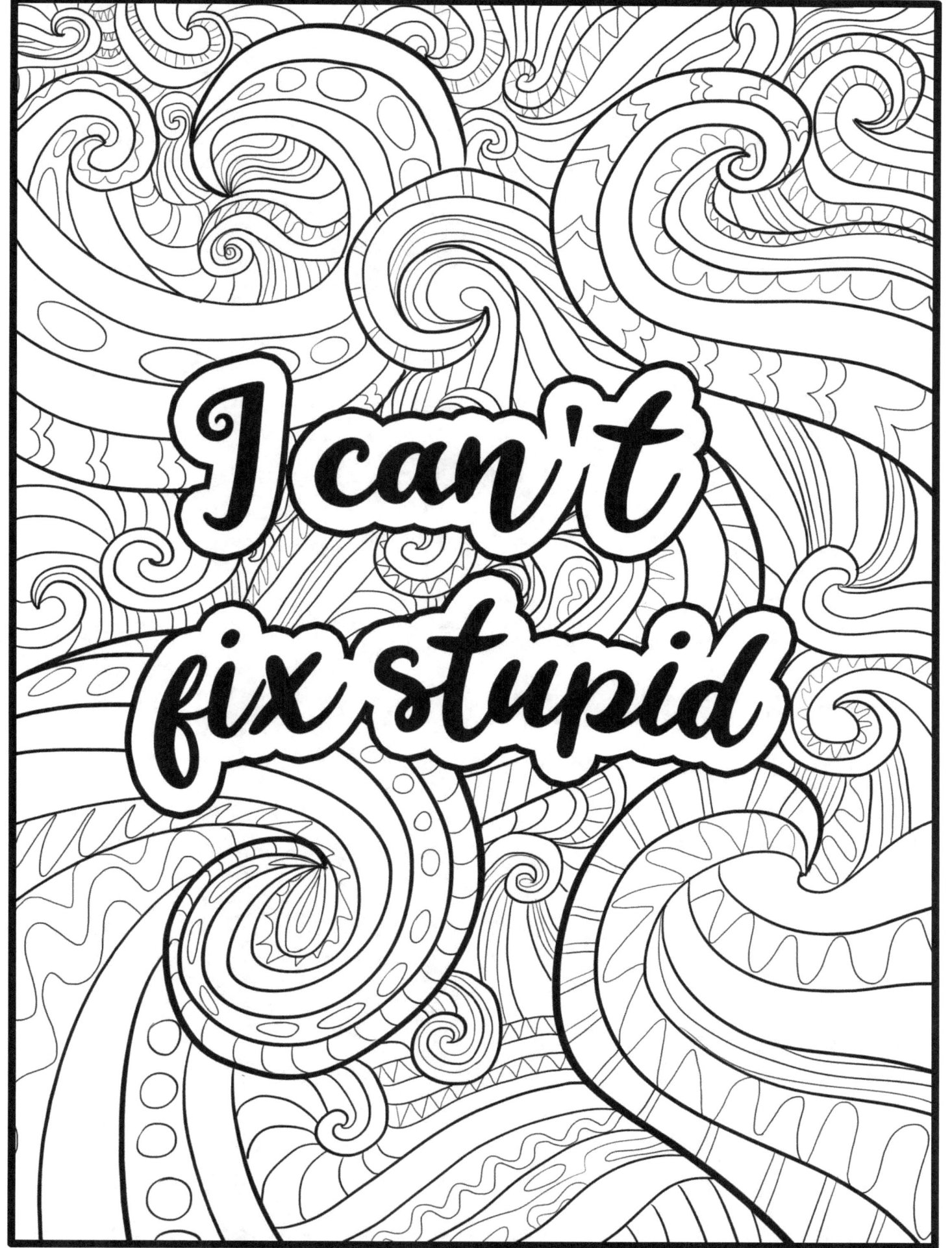

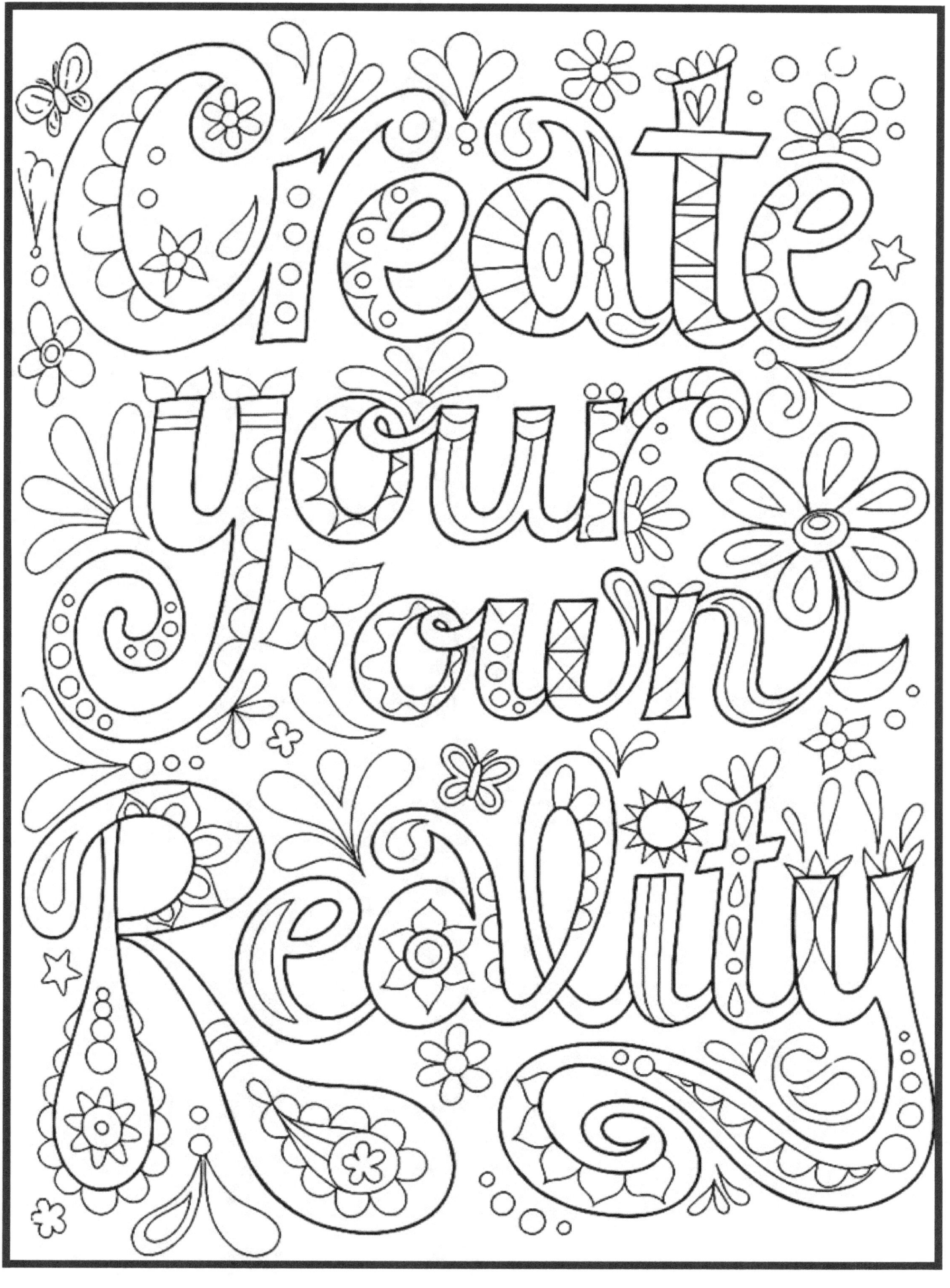

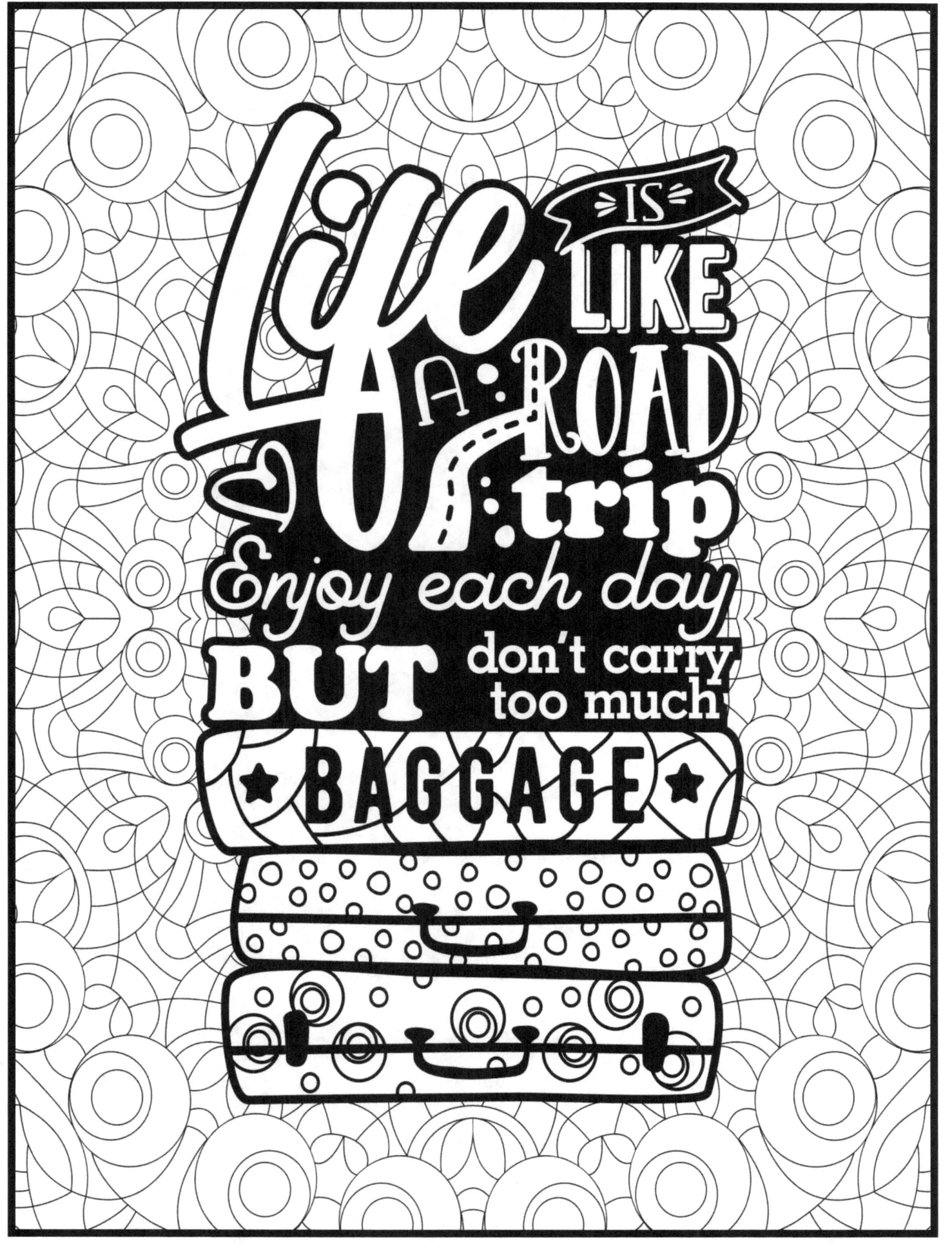

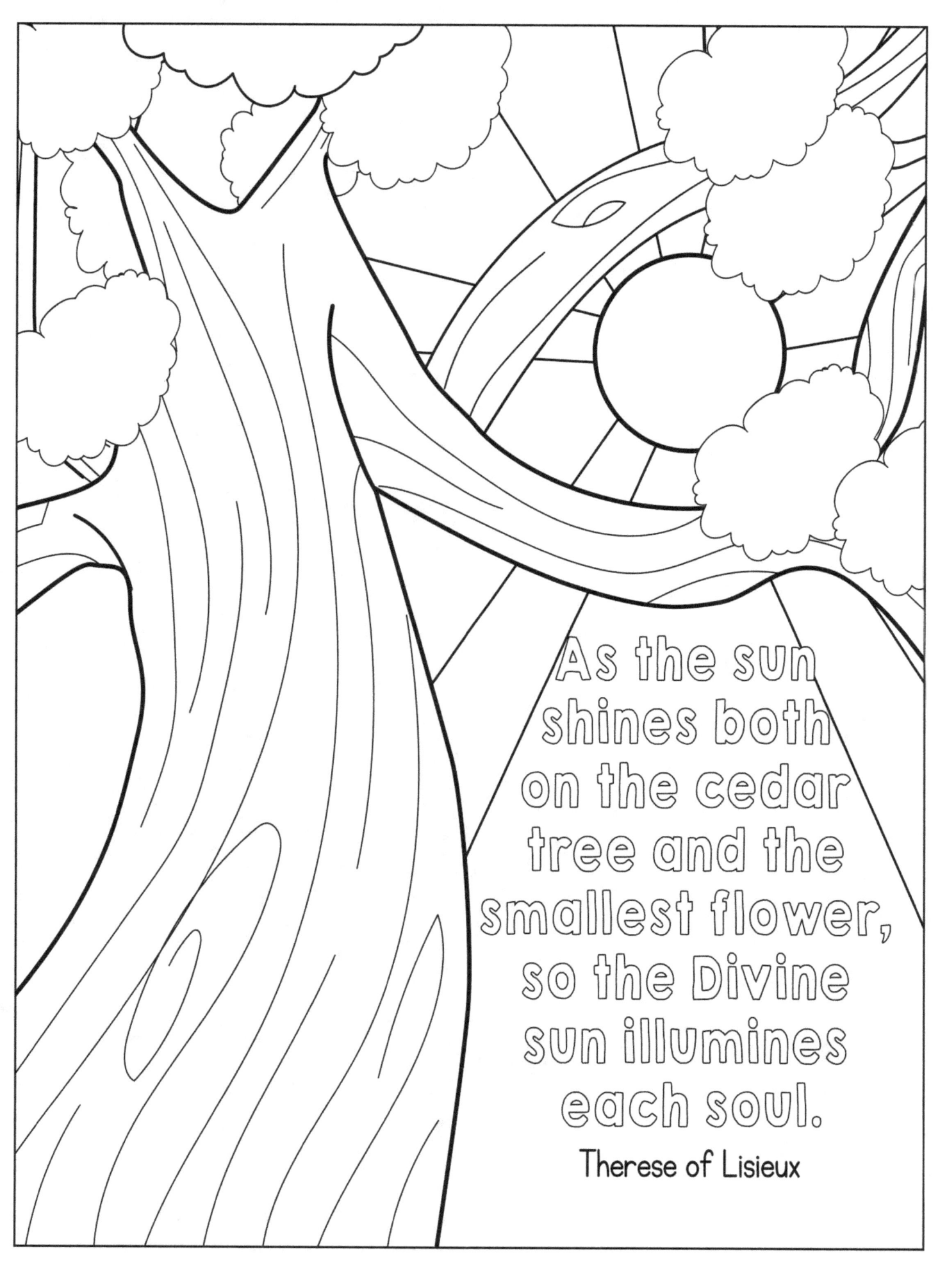

As the sun shines both on the cedar tree and the smallest flower, so the Divine sun illumines each soul.

Therese of Lisieux

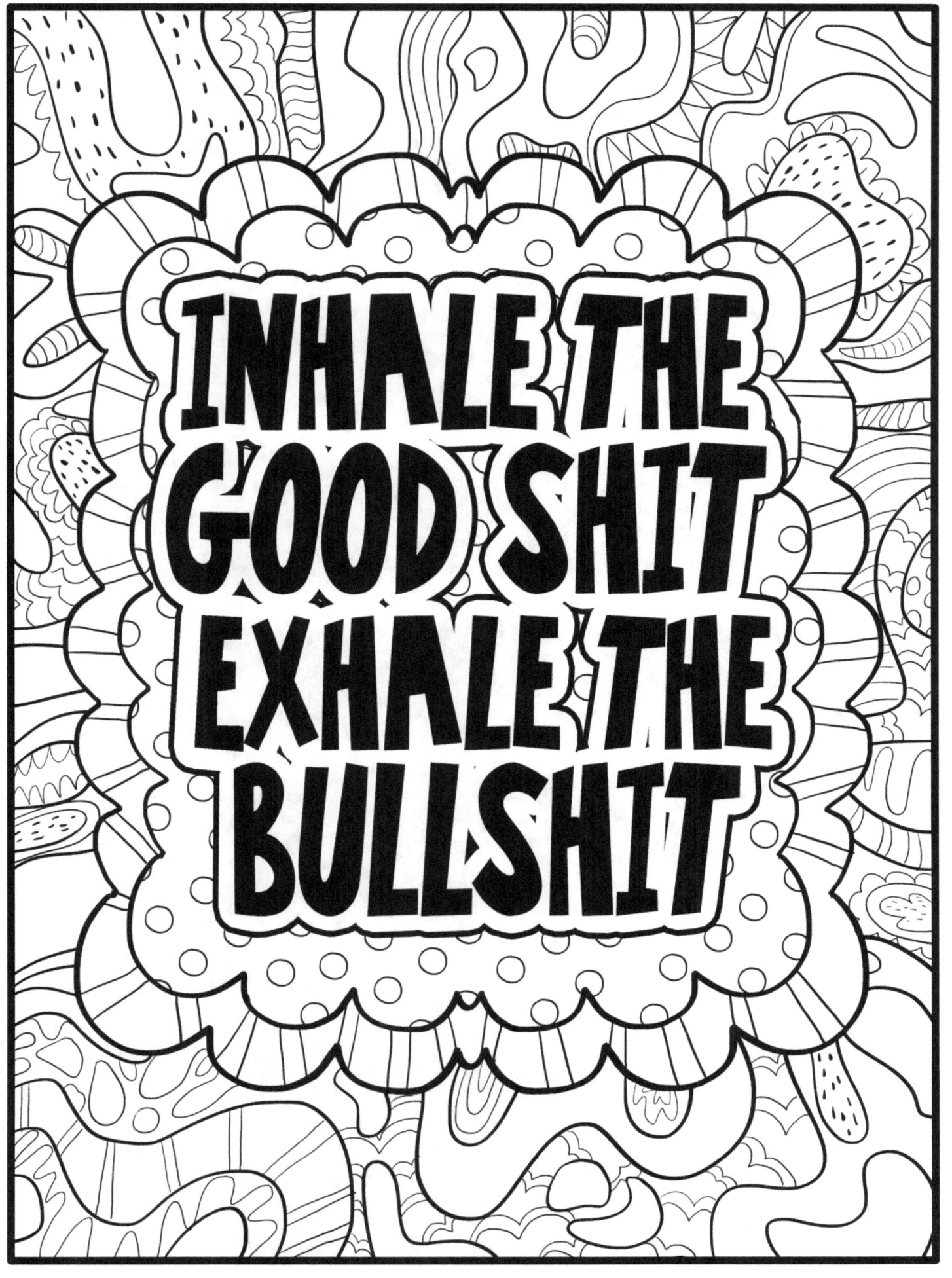

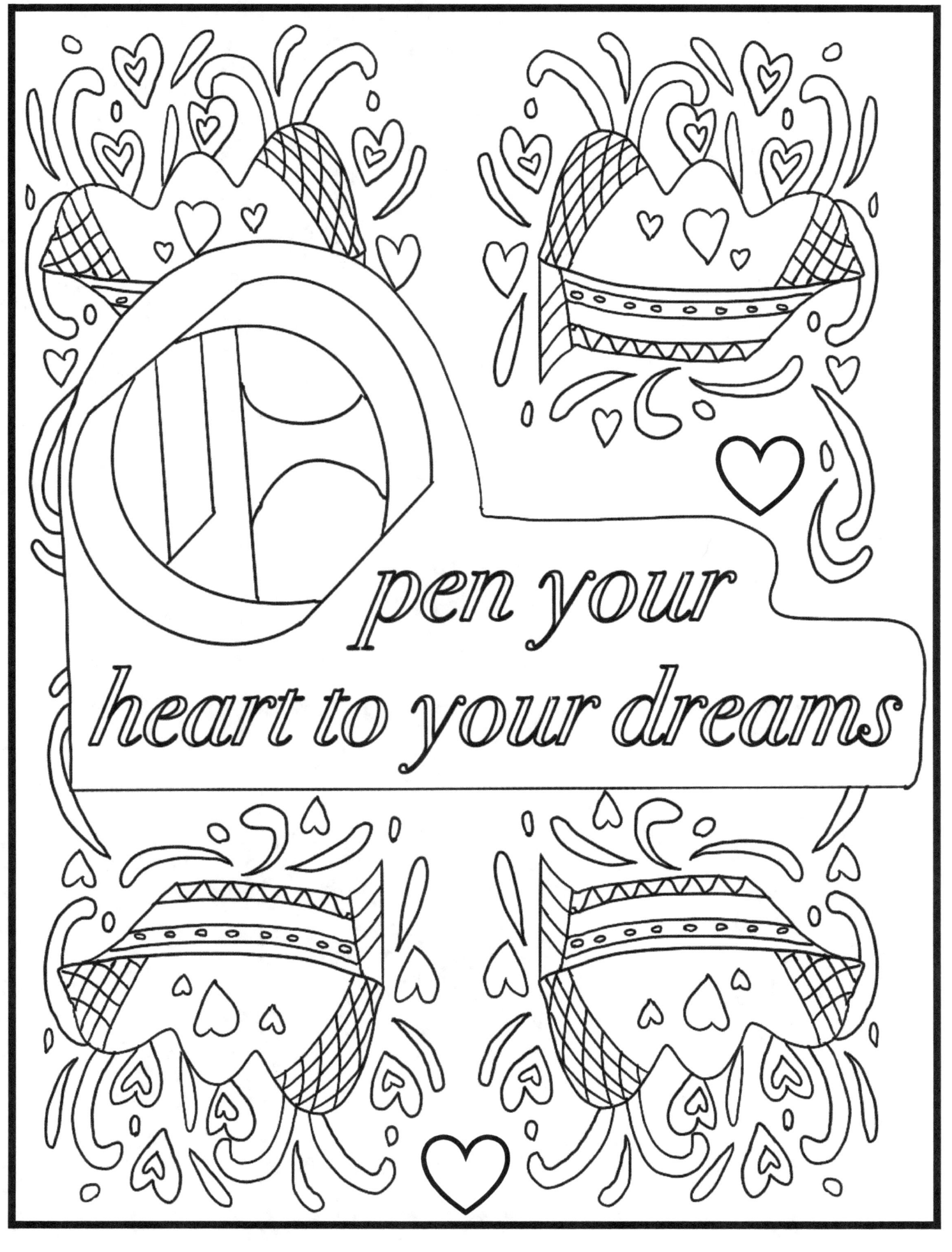

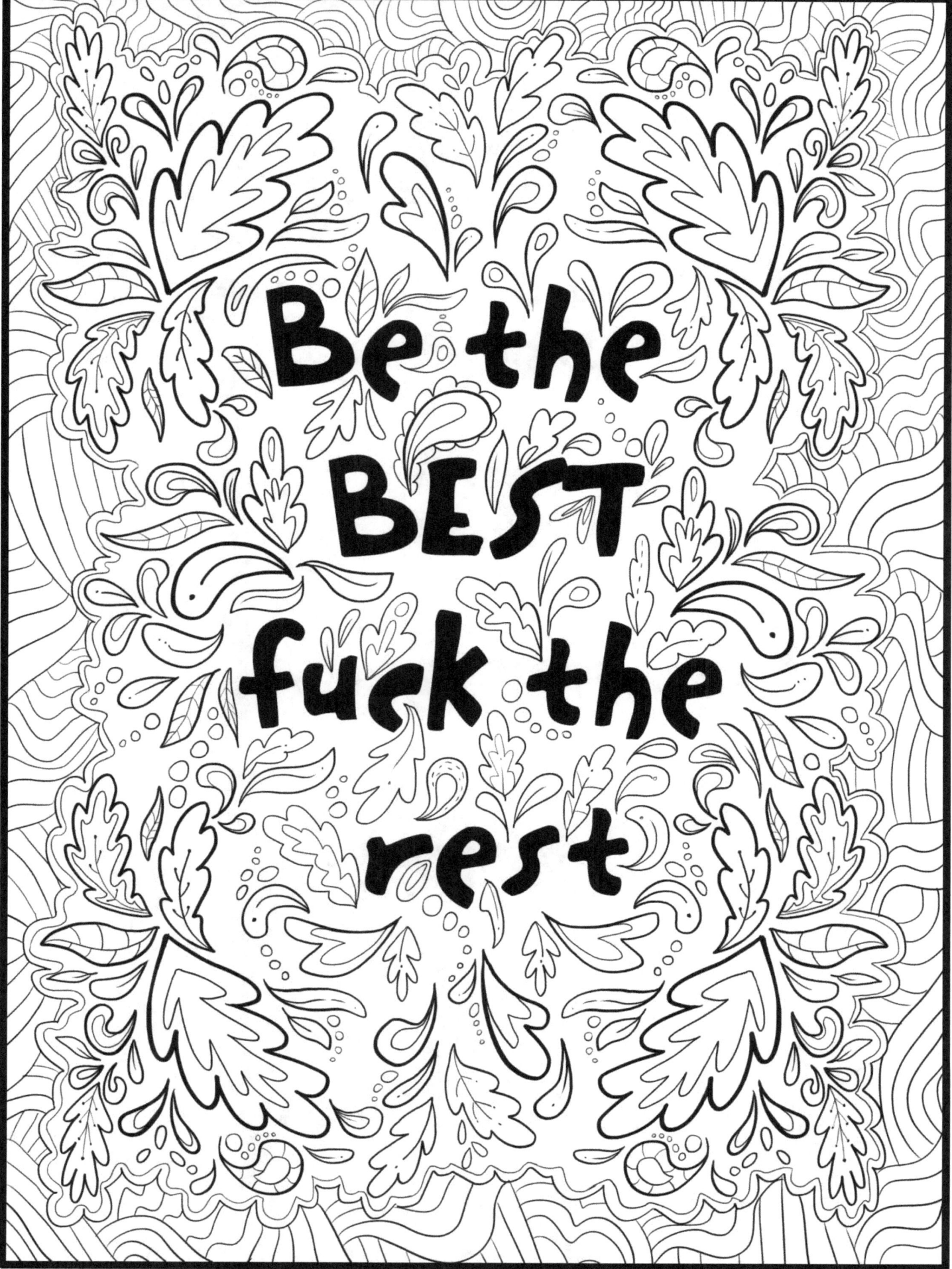

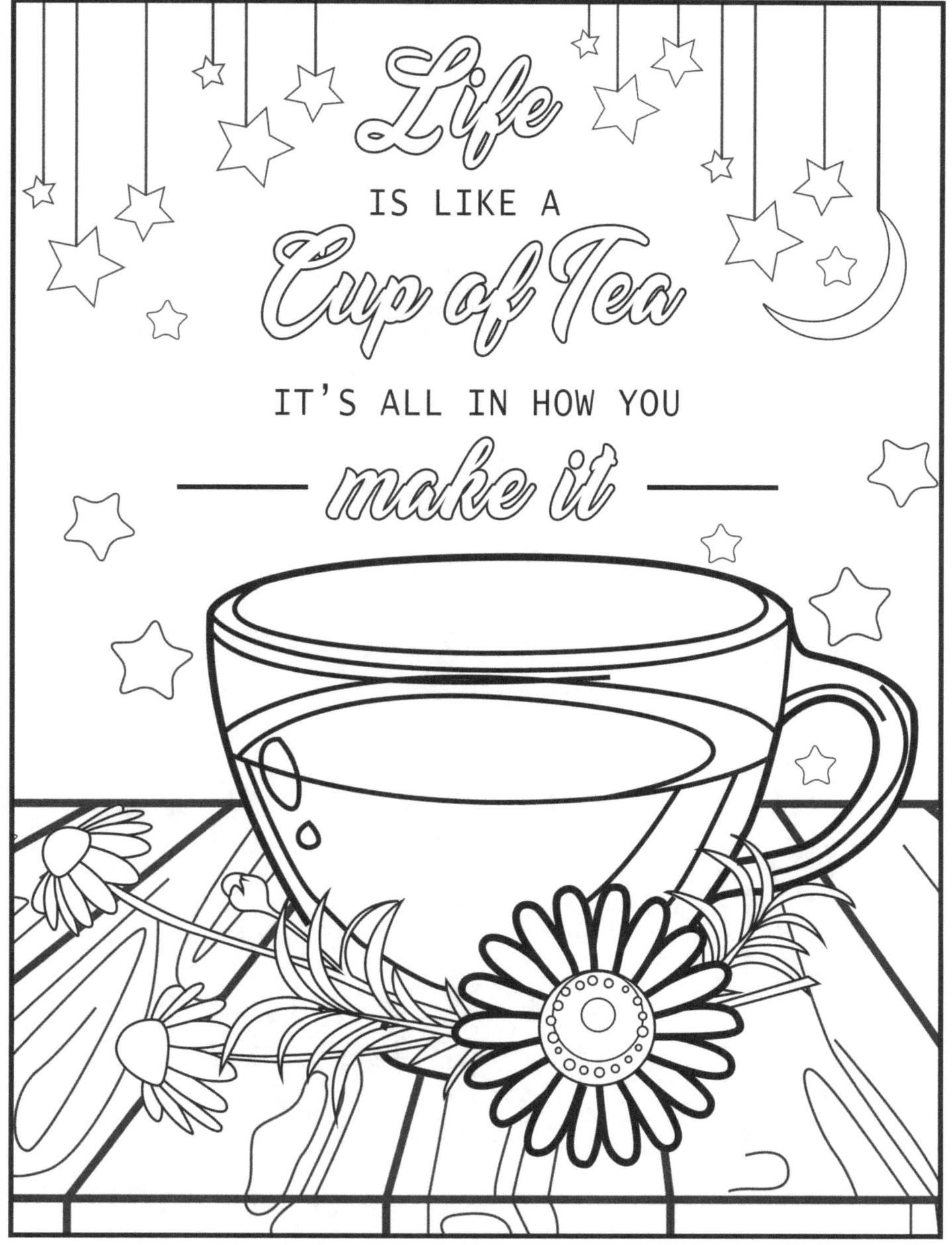

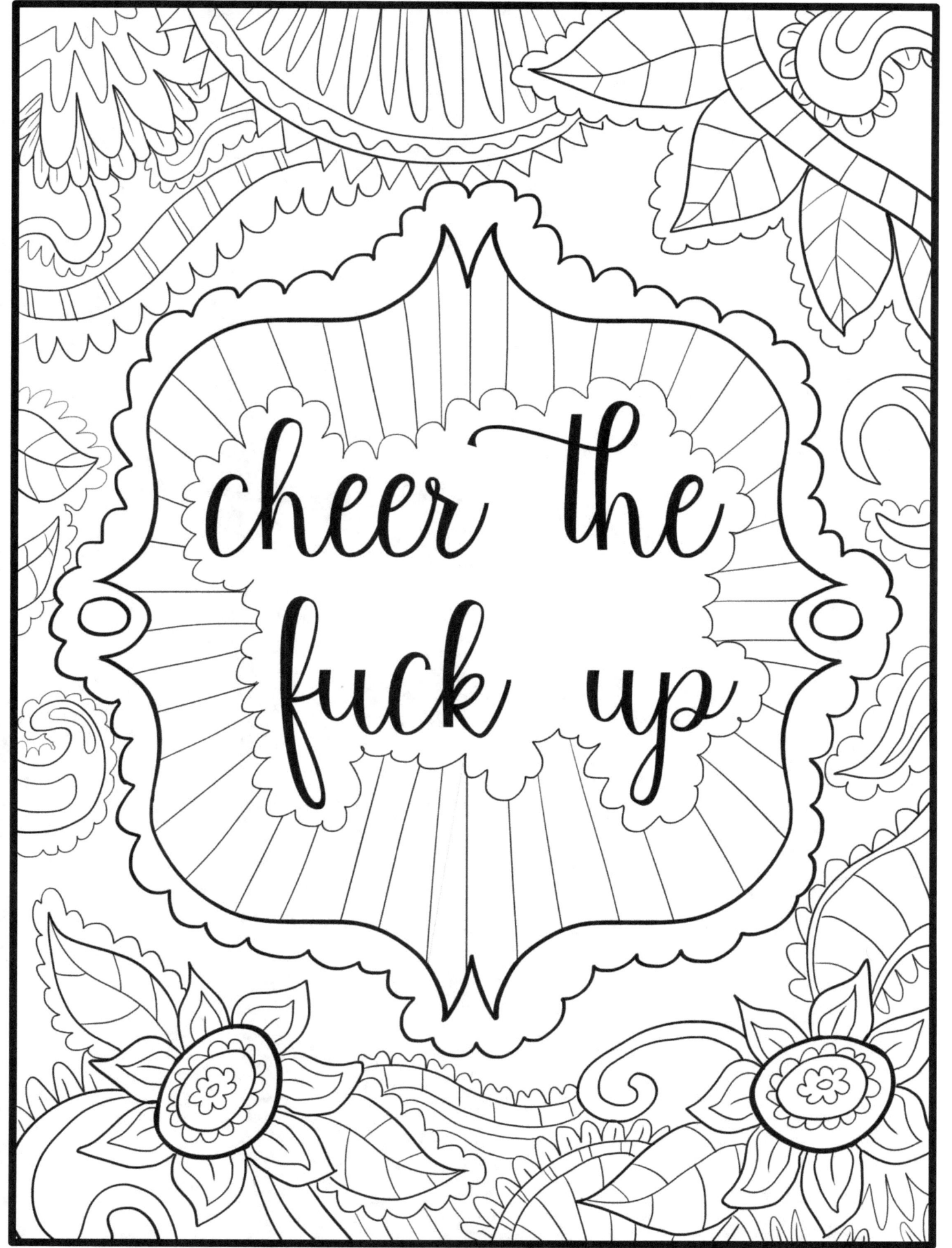

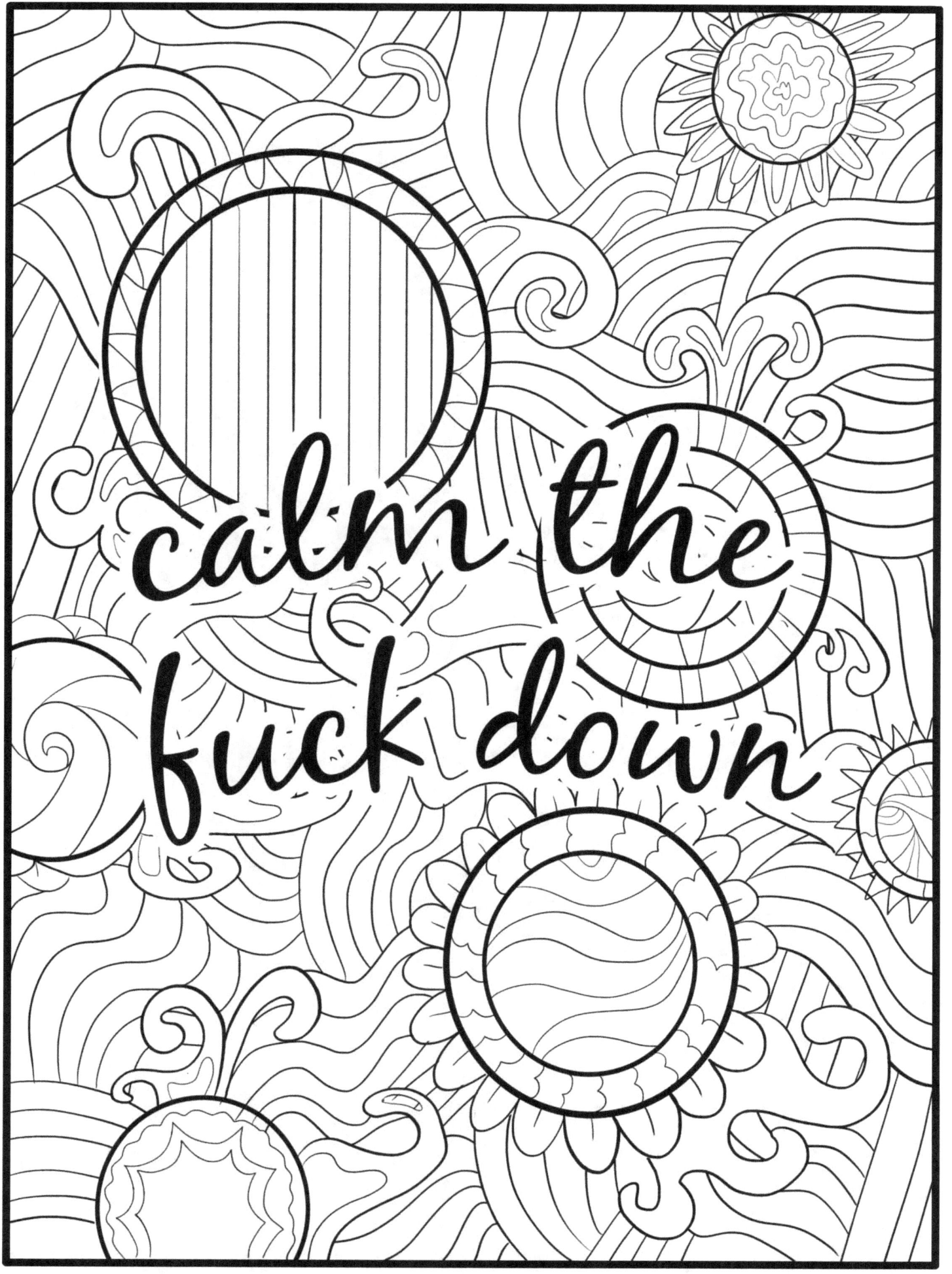

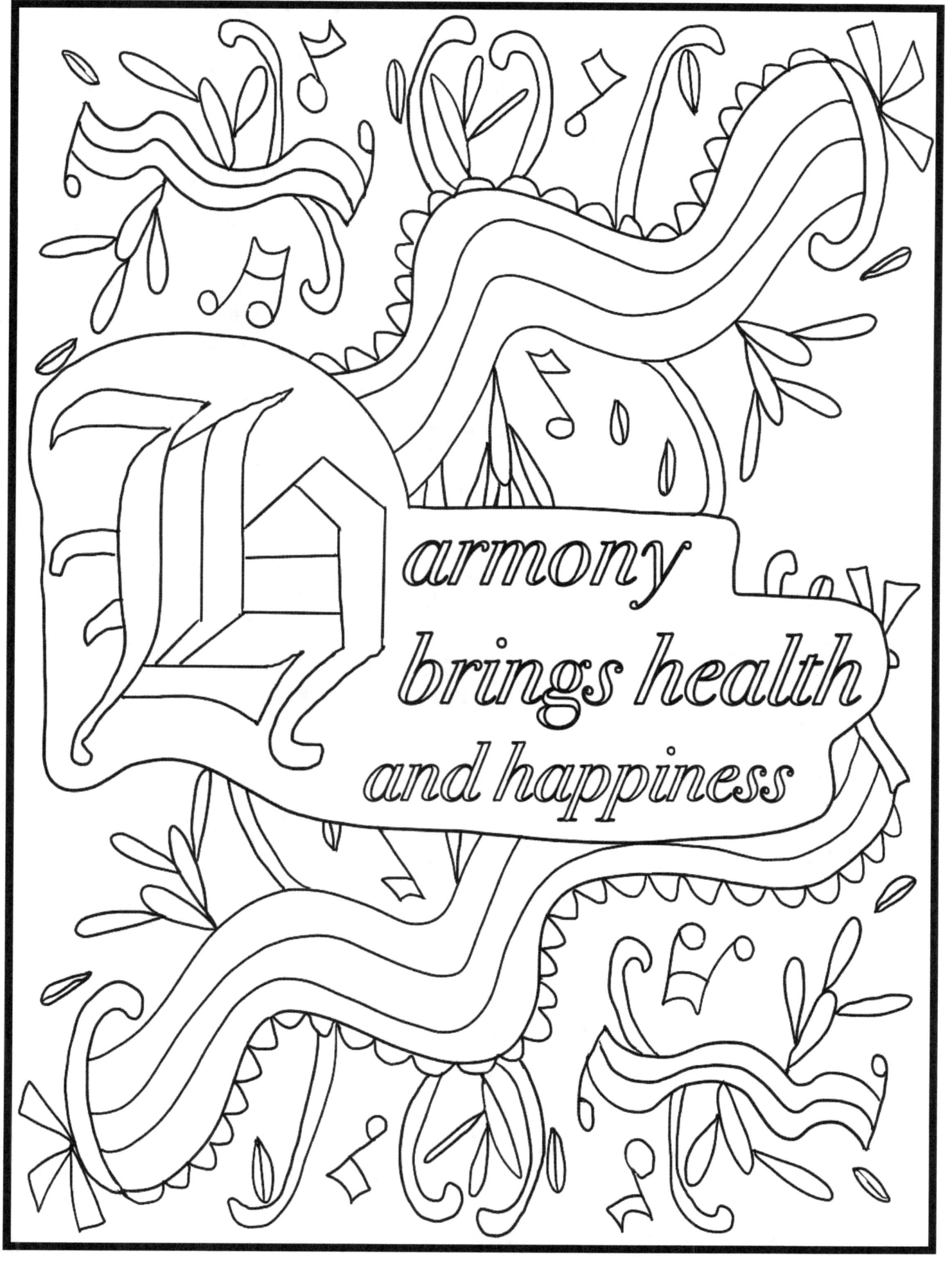

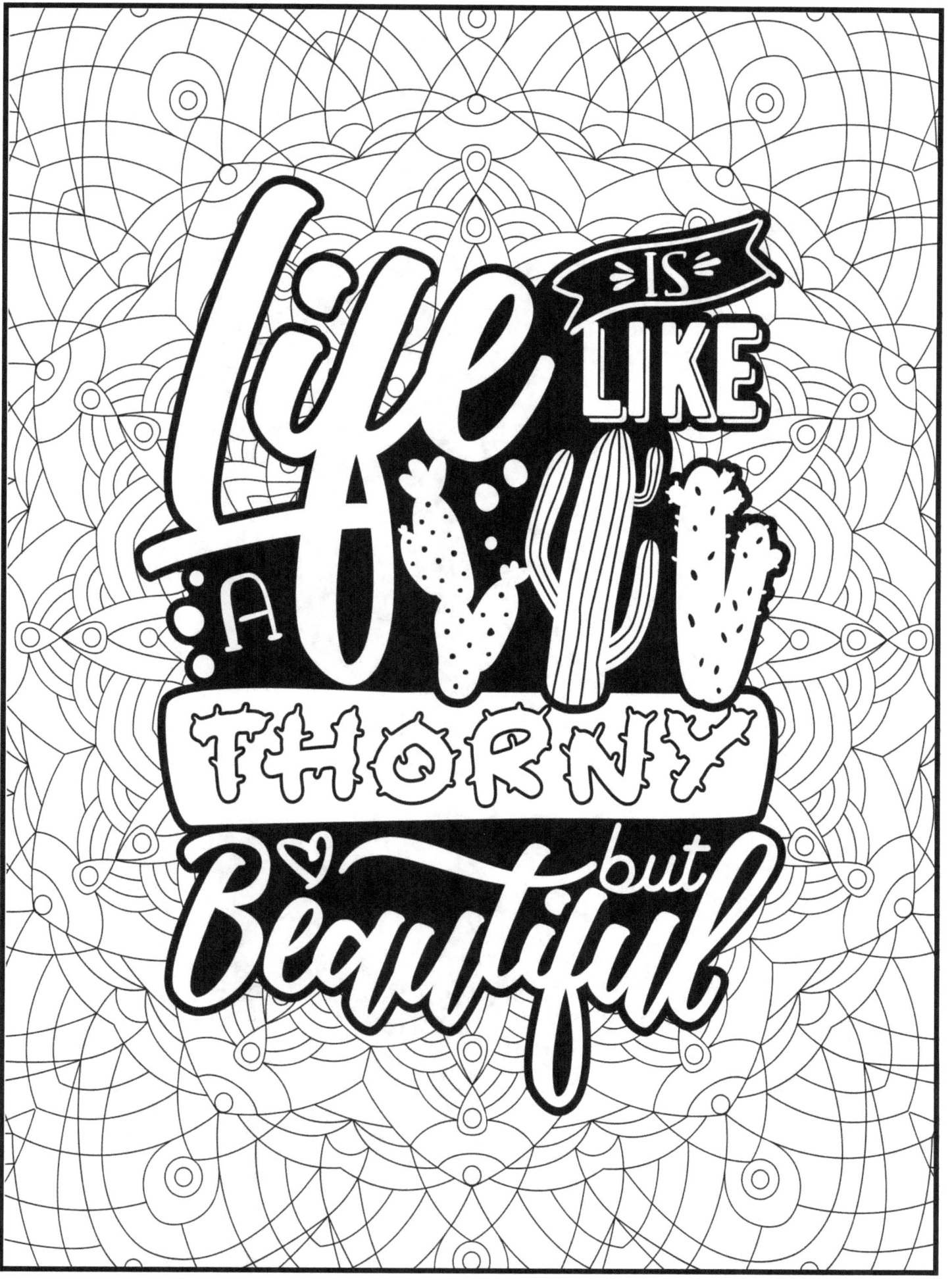